Disclaimer

The Author and Publisher has strived to be as accurate this book, notwithstanding the fact that he does not warr within are accurate due to the rapidly changing nature of the Internet. made to verify information provided in this publication, the Author and Publisher assumes no responsibility for errors, omissions, or contrary interpretation of the subject matter herein. Any perceived slights of specific persons, peoples, or organizations are unintentional. This eBook contains general information about medical conditions and treatments. The information is not medical advice, and should not be treated as such.

Limitation of warranties

The medical information in this eBook is provided "as is" without any representations or warranties, express or implied. *Shingles Health Tips* makes no representations or warranties in relation to the medical information herein.

Without prejudice to the generality of the foregoing paragraph, *Shingles Health Tips* does not warrant that the medical information in this eBook is complete, true, accurate, up-to-date, or non-misleading.

Professional assistance

You must not rely on the information in this eBook as an alternative to medical advice from your doctor or other professional healthcare provider.

If you have any specific questions about any medical matter, you should consult your doctor or other professional healthcare provider.

If you think you may be suffering from any medical condition, you should seek immediately medical attention.

You should never delay seeking medical advice, disregard medical advice, or discontinue medical treatment because of information in this eBook.

Liability

Nothing in this medical disclaimer will limit any of our liabilities in any way that is not permitted under applicable law, or exclude any of our liabilities that may not be excluded under applicable law.

out of date

1 What is Shingles?

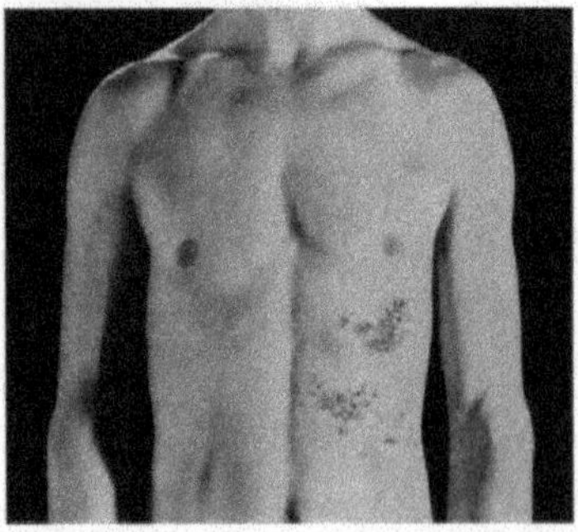

Herpes zoster is a double-stranded DNA virus, a member of the alpha herpes virus family. A century ago, it was generally accepted that herpes zoster shingles did not have any serious health consequences, and it should be treated as such. However, more recent medical research has shown that the course of herpes zoster shingles infection can have adverse consequences on an infected individual for years.

The virus causing chickenpox, herpes zoster, is one and the same as the zoster shingles virus. Varicella, or chickenpox, is an infectious disease caused by the **Varicella-Zoster virus** (VZV), which results in itching, a blister-like rash, tiredness and fever. The zoster virus spreads from one or several ganglia along the nerves of an affected segment and leading to the infection of the corresponding area of skin supplied by the spinal nerve (its dermatome), causing a painful rash. The dermatomes most frequently affected are those of the thorax, abdomen, and ophthalmic branch of the trigeminal nerve. Shown below is an electron micrograph of Varicella zoster (chickenpox) virus, at around 150,000-fold magnification.

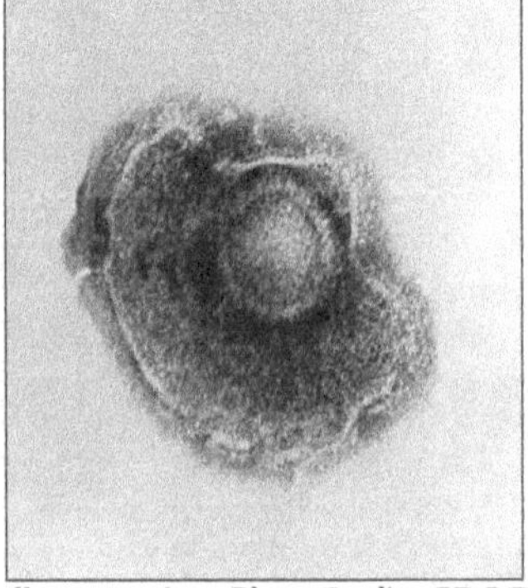

Electron micrograph of Varicella zoster virus. Photo Credit: CDC/Dr. Erskine Palmer/B.G. Partin

Shingles History

The main problem with establishing a link between herpes zoster and chickenpox, and a viral causation of both, is that **there is no animal host on which to do experiments**. This is an infectious disease which can't jump to animals. Thus, much of the evidence confirming a viral cause and mechanism of herpes zoster and chickenpox had to be taken from **clinical and epidemiological observations**. After the link was proven in the 1950's, a live attenuated virus was established in 1974, and acyclovir anti-viral treatment was developed in the 1980's, a tremendous improvement occurred in the prevention and treatment of varicella zoster virus (VZV).

The term "herpes" is generally attributed to Hippocrates and its etymology is derived from the Greek term "to creep." The terms “shingles” or “zoster” both mean “belt,” or a belt-like dermal rash, derived from the Greek term zõstêr. Zõstêr is a reactivation of the latent varicella–zoster virus, usually in the sensory nerve cells. Shingles is caused by the same virus that causes chickenpox (a disease common among young people, which manifests itself through virulent outbursts of itchy blisters all over the body). Pliny, the Greek philosopher, wrote of the difference between herpes simplex and herpes zoster, and accurately described the characteristic appearance of herpes zoster on only one side of the trunk. The term "herpes zoster" was first used to describe the development of vesicular rashes of what is now known to be varicella zoster virus (VZV).

William Heberden, in the late 18th century, found a way to differentiate the clinical features and course of varicella from the clinical features of smallpox. Heberden also saw that those who once had chickenpox "were not capable of having it again." In 1831, Richard Bright suggested herpes zoster arose from the dorsal root ganglion. Felix von Bärensprung confirmed this in 1861. However, only by the start of the 20th century, were the first indications that herpes zoster and chickenpox were caused by the same virus. Post herpetic neuralgia as a consequence of shingles has been known since the early 19th century.

In 1888, **von Bokay** probably was the first to observe the connection between chickenpox and herpes zoster shingles. He saw that household exposure to cases of herpes zoster might lead to cases of chickenpox (varicella) in susceptible children. Nonetheless, many failed to see the connection, and von Bokay’s hypothesis was disputed for more than 60 years.

In 1925, **Kundratitz** demonstrated the transmissibility of an infectious agent. Kundratitz showed that vesicular fluid, taken from a child with chickenpox, when applied to mildly scarred skin of other children not having a prior history of chickenpox, could produce a varicella-like rash in the recipient individual. Next, Kundratitz showed that vesicular fluid, taken from herpes zoster patients, could produce chickenpox when inoculated into susceptible children. Also, these same children could in turn re-transmit chickenpox to a non-inoculated child. Kundratitz thus lent credence to the view that chickenpox and herpes zoster have a common basis.

The American pathologist **Goodpasture** developed cell culture methods using embryonic hen's eggs. He then went on to show that these embryonic hen's eggs cultures could be used to study herpes viruses. Goodpasture, in 1944, took vesicular fluid from herpes zoster lesions and inoculated small biopsies of human skin, which was then grafted onto the membrane of hen's eggs cultures. Days later, the characteristic cytopathology of herpes infection manifested. Goodpasture therefore showed the transmission of infective material from herpes zoster lesions.

That the active principal transmission agent was a virus was first conclusively visualized by **Ruska** in 1948. He demonstrated that the virus particles of both varicella (chickenpox) and herpes zoster were identical in appearance and size, when viewed under the electron microscope. Additionally, electron microscopy enabled the actual virus structure to be understood.

The final proof that the varicella chickenpox virus and the herpes zoster shingles virus were identical appeared in 1952. **Weller and Stoddard** presented serum isolates from either varicella or zoster to roller cultures of human tissue. Identical cytopathology was observed from either varicella or zoster vesicle fluid. Weller utilized experimental evidence to conclude that both varicella and herpes zoster are caused by one and only one virus, which Weller called "varicella zoster virus" (VZV). In 1954, Weller and Coons presented hard evidence that the chickenpox virus and the herpes zoster shingles virus are one and the same.

In 1986, molecular genetics techniques allowed the complete DNA sequence of VZV to be determined. VZV was found to be a linear, double-stranded DNA virus, approximately 100,000 base pairs long, with close analogies to the herpes simplex type-1 virus family.

While all this viral identification work was in progress, advances in the understanding of the human pathogenesis of herpes zoster were occurring. Starting with Richard Bright in 1831, then later with von Bärensprung in 1861, a correspondence between the herpes zoster lesions and the underlying peripheral nerve distribution was noticed. Von Bärensprung also demonstrated, at autopsy, damage in the corresponding dorsal root ganglion for a patient who had died from a case of acute herpes zoster.

Then, in 1900, **Head and Campbell** published a detailed study of post-mortem pathology of several individuals who had suffered from various stages of herpes zoster before death. In every case, there was pronounced pathology in the posterior root ganglion supplying the area of skin around the shingles rash. The pathological changes extended to the nerve roots and spinal cord tracts. Significantly, these pathological changes developed over time after the onset of a herpes zoster rash. Head and Campbell were able to create a map revealing the dermatomal distribution of sensory nerves.

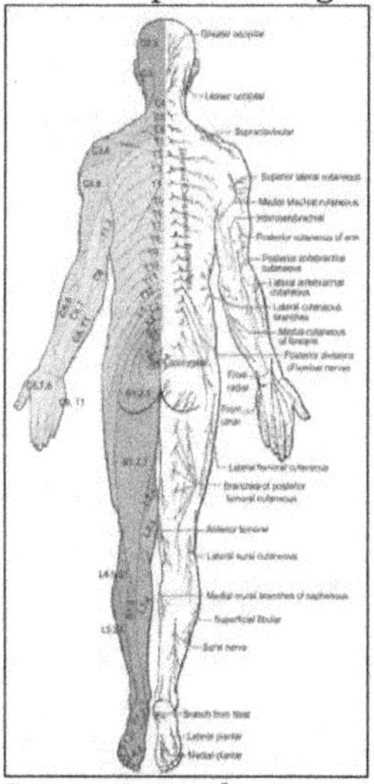

Dermatomes and cutaneous nerves. Credit: Wikipedia (Dermatome (anatomy))

Several researchers, including **Joseph Garland**, hinted that, like herpes simplex virus, herpes zoster might be a re-activation of the latent form of the virus that originally caused the varicella (chickenpox) outbreak. In 1964, in a bold hypothesis, **Edgar Hope-Simpson** put forward the idea that herpes zoster manifests itself as an individual's immunity to VZV is weakened. This hypothesis was drawn from 16 years of epidemiological experience as a general practitioner in England. Earlier, Hope-Simpson had proven that varicella (chickenpox) could be acquired from herpes zoster but not vice versa. In Hope-Simpson's epidemiology study, the incidence rates of herpes zoster increased steadily with age. Overall, the incidence was 3-4 per 1000 persons per year. Hope-Simpson confirmed that:

1. zoster could not be acquired from other cases of zoster
2. zoster could not be acquired from varicella (chickenpox)
3. zoster did not occur as an epidemic

Hope-Simpson's hypothesis is as follows:

1. during the primary infection, the virus entered sensory nerve endings and was transported centrally to the sensory ganglion
2. once transported to the sensory ganglion, VZV established latency, and stayed "under the radar," evading immune surveillance
3. reactivation of VZV could occur intermittently, but the immune system kept VZV in check
4. At some point, immunity falls below a threshold level, allowing reactivation of the infectious virus
5. once reactivated, VZV could multiply and pass down the sensory nerve to the skin

Subsequent experimental proof of the Hope-Simpson hypothesis was demonstrated using immunofluorescence and electron microscopy, showing the exact site of the latency of VZV in a sensory ganglion. At autopsy, VZV DNA and RNA were obtained within sensory ganglia from individuals who had recent outbreaks of either chickenpox or herpes zoster. The Hope-Simpson hypothesis has withstood the test of time, nearly 50 years after its introduction. Cellular immune control is now known to be the mitigating factor in determining whether VZV reactivates or not.

Some of the important advances in mankind's understanding of the varicella zoster virus are shown in the accompanying table.

Year	Event	Reference
1888	Suggestion of a relationship between chickenpox and herpes zoster	Von Bokay
1925	The transmissibility of a varicella infectious agent demonstrated	Kundratitz
1943	"Ramsay Hunt" syndrome ascribed to herpes zoster	Garland
1948	Electron microscopy visualization of VZV	Ruska
1952	isolation of varicella virus from clinical cases	Weller and Stod
1958	Final conclusion both chickenpox and herpes zoster caused by a common virus, officially termed VZV	Weller, et al
1964	An hypothesis on the reactivation of the latent form of VZV	Hope-Simpso
1974	Attenuated live vaccine developed	Takahishi, et a
1980's	Aciclovir developed as a treatment for VZV infection	
1986	Complete determination of VZV DNA sequence	Davison and Sc
1997	Varicella vaccine used to reduce herpes zoster severity	Redman, et a

Table 1: A broad history of Varicella zoster understanding

The 1950's saw another turning point in the history of herpes zoster shingles. Medical science came to an understanding that the disease was not as benign as originally believed. While children or young adults might not be severely affected by herpes zoster shingles, the risks of contracting the shingles disease increase with age. In addition, with age, the risks of the illness becoming severe increase significantly. After researchers discovered the potential health threat of herpes zoster shingles, investment in medical research towards a shingles cure has significantly increased. Since the 1950's, it has become evident that over 25% of adults over 40 will contract shingles, and that the chances of a person developing herpes zoster shingles increase with age. Although herpes zoster shingles usually affects the middle-aged to elderly, even younger individuals can develop herpes zoster.

There is one final significant entry in the history of mankind's understanding of VZV, and that is the **acute treatment of VZV**. The first anti-viral used was adenosine arabinoside (vidarabine), which required hospitalization to administer. Even still, it was difficult to administer, and toxicity was a problem. Then, in the 1980's, acicycloir was discovered and developed. Both oral and intravenous applications have been developed, and they represent a significant improvement in therapy. Acyclovir has become the chosen drug to treat VZV.

Hope-Simpson's hypothesis by now is well established, but lesser known is his views on the evolution of VZV. Hope-Simpson believed the VZV virus evolved its latency strategy to perpetuate itself in small, isolated bands of humans, typical of early stages in human evolution. The basic idea was that VZV hid in adults until a new generation of susceptible hosts was available. The dizzying pace of recent developments in VZV research includes studies of the molecular biology of the VZV genome.

By doing the same sort of genetic analysis as was done on the human mitochondrial genome, and mapping genome changes in various VZV strains, it has been shown the geographical pattern of mutations in the VZV genome matches changes in the human mitochondrial genome, leading to the inference the VZV genome has accompanied man for several hundred thousand years, if not longer. Possibly VZV originated 60 million years ago in African primates, leading to the suggestion that VZV has been handed down to us from our early Australopithecine forebears.

2 The course of the Shingles Disease

Shingles disease is caused by a herpetic virus called Varicella-Zoster Virus (VZV). A key characteristic of herpetic viruses is their ability to lay dormant if the body's immune system is healthy. When infected with the Varicella-Zoster Virus, a patient will develop chickenpox. Once that disease has run its course, the virus remains in the body. It remains dormant in the patient's nervous system and will become inactive for an undefined period. The following table outlines the VZV status during the several stages of Varicella zoster infection in humans.

Disease status:	Never had chickenpox	Had chickenpox	Has Shingles
VZV status:	Does not have ZVZ	Has dormant VZV	Has active VZV

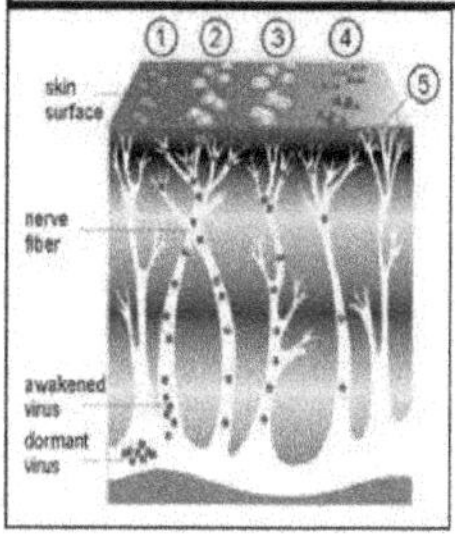

Shingles Infectivity

The Varicella-Zoster Virus is extremely infectious. More than 90% of the United States population has been infected with this virus. In addition, if you live in an environment with individuals infected with Varicella-Zoster Virus, there is a 90% probability that you will be infected as well. Fortunately, in the vast majority of people infected, individuals only develop the initial condition caused by the virus, and that is the chickenpox disease (or Varicella). All herpes simplex viruses are spread by contact, as the virus is shed in tears, saliva and genital secretions. One common form of herpes simplex viral infection results from a kiss given to a child or adult from a person who is in the stage of shedding the Varicella Zoster virus. After the initial stage of infection, the virus then establishes latency in the craniospinal ganglia, a major nervous system structure.

We are still unsure about the mechanism; but as an individual ages, their immune system will gradually become weaker. Moreover, when the immune system is weak enough, the Varicella-Zoster virus (VZV) can travel along the nerves and manifest itself in the form of herpes zoster shingles.

VZV Transmission

Most viruses have a tendency to be more active during certain times of the year. The Varicella-Zoster virus however is not one of them, as it has no seasonal preferences. Case studies have shown that climate also has little to do with the rate at which the virus is transmitted, as it is equally active in all parts of the world. The Varicella-Zoster virus can be transmitted from person to person in two ways:

1. In the majority of cases, through direct contact with one of the exposed sores (the itchy blisters caused by chickenpox).
2. In the minority of cases, through the air, when a person inhales aerosols from an infected person.

VZV Incubation period

The Varicella-Zoster virus has an incubation period of about five to seven days. In that time, it will remain in the lungs, without causing any symptoms or harm. Most commonly, patients experience one or two days of itching, numbness, and throbbing or stabbing pain in the area where the skin lesions appear eventually. After this, it will travel from the lungs throughout the body and it will eventually find its way to the skin. This will take around twelve to fourteen days, after which an individual will start to experience the first symptoms of chickenpox. A typical chickenpox outbreak is shown in the photo below.

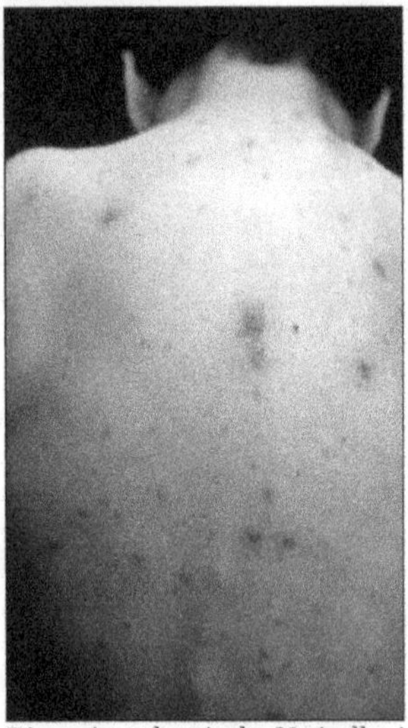

Disseminated vesicular Varicella simplex (chickenpox) rash on a child. Courtesy Wikimedia Commons

Once the chickenpox is treated, the VZV virus will lay dormant for years in the body's sensory ganglia, from which it can reactivate itself to cause herpes zoster shingles. It is this feature of the virus that makes it one of the most resilient viruses around. It allows the Varicella-Zoster virus to survive indefinitely, even if the infected person is not susceptible to chickenpox anymore. In addition, it can reactivate itself multiple times. There are many documented cases of people who have suffered from shingles disease on more than one occasion. Once you have been infected with the Varicella-Zoster Virus, there's no telling if, when or how many times you may have an additional shingles outbreak. Fortunately, in the vast majority of cases, this does not occur.

3 Shingles Symptoms

Although the same virus is involved, shingles symptoms are very different from chickenpox symptoms.

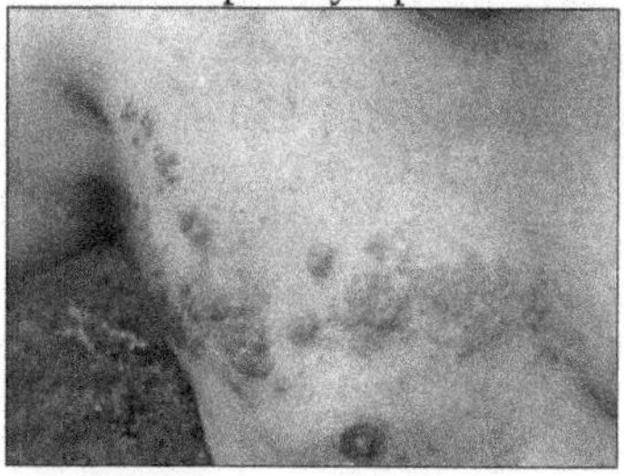

Chickenpox Symptoms

With chickenpox, the most well known symptom is the itchy, red blisters that can appear on the entire surface of the body. In addition, chickenpox symptoms may also include fever, body aches, nausea, loss of appetite and headaches. These symptoms are highly flu-like in nature and will usually manifest themselves before the appearance of the rash. Unless a rash occurs, the illness is very easily mistaken for the flu and people have a tendency to defer a visit to the doctor. This may have serious consequences, as improper treatment could lead to severe complications.

Shingles Symptoms

Shingles symptoms are **quite different** than chickenpox and can be much more serious. Shingles rash, unlike chickenpox, usually **appears on only one side of the midline of the body**. This symptom is characteristic of shingles, and is now known to be the external manifestation of an activation of the Herpes zoster virus as it travels to the patch of skin served by one of the ganglionic nerves.

Here are some common symptoms that individuals experience in the first few days of a shingles episode:

1. drooping eyelids
2. chills and fevers
3. genital lesions
4. headaches
5. loss of hearing
6. pain in joints
7. limited full eye movement
8. glands become swollen
9. difficulty moving facial muscles
10. vision and taste problems.
11. abdomen pain

The first sign of herpes zoster shingles is pain. You will start to feel mild to excruciating pain in the affected area. Note that the pain will usually only be felt on one side of your body. Besides the pain, the same area may be affected by burning, tingling or numbness. This is why the medical condition of shingles may be mistaken with heart, lung or kidney disease (depending upon the location of the pain). This pain usually appears only with adult patients. Juvenile shingles is often pain-free.

Other than the pain, the most important symptom of shingles is also the most obvious, and that is the **shingles rash**. The rash can appear anytime from 1 day to 3 weeks after the initial symptoms and it is usually located on the chest and upper back. Although the torso is usually the affected area, herpes zoster shingles can also appear on the face, neck, eyes and other body parts. The shingles rash usually takes the shape of a stripe or belt, a fact that differentiates it from other rashes. It is unlikely that you will suffer from a disease other than shingles if your rash has this particular shape. The rash contains blisters, which are filled with serous exudates. This rash is often similar to that of chickenpox, but **it is more localized**. Note that sometimes shingles can occur without a rash. The condition is called "*zoster sine herpete*". Shingles are blister-like vesicles that look like a case of chickenpox, only these vesicles are smaller. Shingles appears in clusters that develop within a week's time of the onset of symptoms.

During the active infection phase, Varicella zoster virus (VZV) inflames the nervous ganglia and destroys nerve endings. The result of this viral attack is frequently **post-herpetic neuralgia** (PHN), a residual pain syndrome from shingles and shingle's most common complication.

Other Shingles symptoms

Shingles disease also presents a series of other symptoms, which can be equally serious. Among them are fatigue, body aches, abdominal pain, joint pain and swollen lymph nodes. In 10% to 25% of the cases, the rash can appear near the eyes and ears, a situation in which symptoms such as trouble moving facial muscles, a drooping eyelid, eye motion loss, hearing loss, and problems with taste and sight may appear. In addition, there are a few cases in which reported symptoms include keratitis, conjunctivitis, optic nerve palsies, vertigo and uveitis. These unusual symptoms, characterized by two particular outcomes of shingles, stand out. These two are termed herpes zoster *ophthalmicus* and herpes zoster *oticus*.

4 Shingles Medical Diagnosis

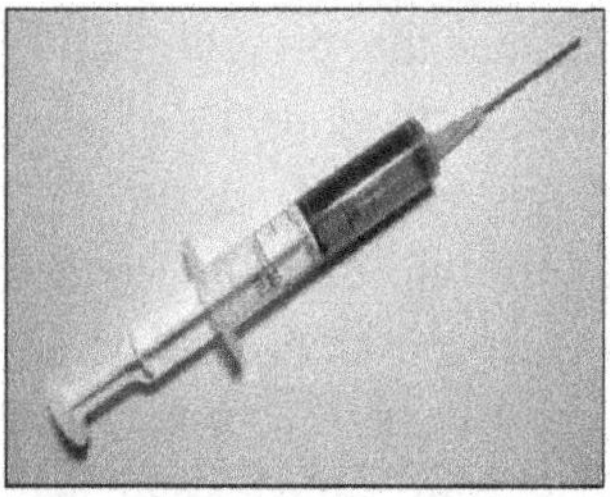

Several methods can be used to diagnose shingles. Correctly diagnosing herpes zoster shingles is of paramount importance, because the wrong treatment may have unwanted consequences. Once the shingles rash has appeared, diagnosing shingles becomes relatively easy, as the rash pattern is very specific. This rash pattern is unique to shingles. Only one other type of herpetic virus (herpes simplex virus) can manifest itself through a similar type of rash, and that rarely happens. With the rash present, you can be virtually certain that you are suffering from herpes zoster shingles, but a full physical examination and a complete medical history will still be necessary in order to be 100% sure of a shingles diagnosis.

Shingles can be harder to diagnose in some cases. If the rash has not appeared yet, or a few weeks have already passed and the rash is gone, a 100% shingles diagnosis will be harder to obtain. This is also the case with "zoster sine herpete." When the rash is not present, you need to verify shingles with a series of laboratory tests. While reaching a shingles diagnosis may be difficult and tedious, its importance trumps any technical diagnostic difficulty in comparison. Misdiagnosis may have potentially fatal consequences.

Laboratory and diagnostic tests

The most commonly used laboratory test detects the presence of IgM antibody in your blood. This particular antibody only appears when the patient has been infected with the Varicella-Zoster virus. In addition, the antibody appears only when the virus is active, so it will only be detected if the patient is suffering from chickenpox or herpes zoster shingles disease. If the virus is present in the body but is in its dormant state, this antibody will not appear. In more advanced laboratories, a sample from a blister can also be taken and then used with polymerase chain reaction (PCR) methods or an electron microscope to detect the Varicella-Zoster Virus.

Cell culture of Varicella Zoster virus. Photo courtesy of Dr. Linda Stannard, University of Cape Town, SA, and Virology Laboratory of the Yale-New Haven Hospital.

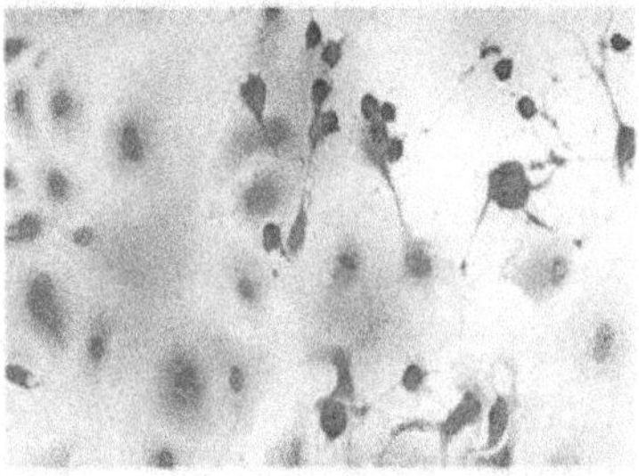

Diagnostic tests for shingles are very specific and quite accurate, so if there is the possibility of shingles, these tests will be able to definitely offer a diagnosis. **Scrapings of a shingles lesion, and subsequent cytology, are typically performed to confirm the diagnosis of shingles**. Shown below is a typical cell culture of VZV, with associated cell ballooning.

5 Shingles Treatment

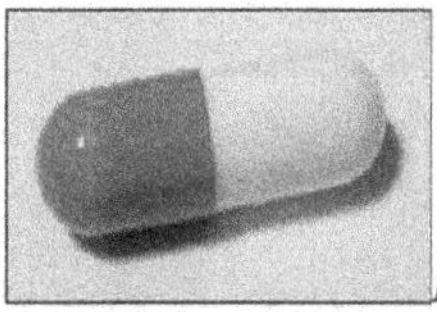

As the severity of herpes zoster shingles in adults became more and more apparent to medical scientists, the importance of finding an effective treatment also became evident.

Over the last 70 years, medicine has taken huge steps forward, and we now have many effective ways to deal with shingles. Unfortunately, a way to eliminate the Varicella-Zoster virus from the body is elusive, but with proper care and treatment, one can shorten healing time and greatly enhance the quality of life of a herpes zoster shingles patient.

As a first line of precaution, **you should go to your hospital's emergency department** if you experience any of the following:

- If you feel sick or have a high fever
- Redness, pain, or rash (with or without blisters) on the face, **especially near your eyes**
- If shingles blisters persist and spread to other parts of the body

As the virus cannot be eliminated, and the rash cannot go away on its own, the therapeutic focus for shingles treatments is to alleviate the pain. The primary weapon against pain is analgesic drugs. Analgesics are drugs that are engineered specifically to act on a person's nervous system and make the pain go away. Unfortunately, not all analgesics work for shingles pain. For example, Ibuprofen will do little, even against the mid-range pain of a herpes zoster shingles patient.

Analgesics

For severe shingles pain, doctors will often prescribe morphine, and while it may be extremely effective, morphine is not without its side effects. Morphine is classified as an opiate analgesic and it can help patients with even the most debilitating pain.

Unfortunately, morphine is extremely addictive, so small doses are recommended. Frequently, patients with shingles become addicted to morphine. If that happens, the pain from shingles disease will seem minor compared to the complications of morphine addiction. When a patient addicted to morphine stops taking it, drug withdrawal takes place, and it can be lethal for patients with heart or lung disease, or neurologically unhealthy. Even for relatively healthy patients, morphine withdrawal has awful symptoms like vomiting, frequent diarrhea, painful involuntary ejaculation, insomnia, high blood pressure, and an increase in white blood cell count, muscle twitches, hot and cold flashes, anxiety, tachycardia and many others. Morphine should only be used for the extreme cases of herpes zoster shingles pain, and it will offer the patient shingles relief, but the side effects are enormous.

For more mild cases of shingles pain, Calamine is a very good analgesic lotion. It can offer a patient much-needed relief from shingles pain, and it can also act as a mild antiseptic, therefore, it can stop the burst blisters from being infected and causing infections. If Calamine lotion is used, apply it liberally to any shingles lesions. If shingles lesions are widespread and severe, consider applying a wet dressing. A drying therapy, such as an air-loss bed or oxygen, and Silvadene ointment, may be used as well.

Another analgesic solution is a cream that contains capsaicin. However, this should only be used after the blisters have formed a crust. Other analgesics that have proven their effectiveness against shingles pain are lidocaine and gabapentin.

Antivirals

Besides an analgesic, an antiviral should also be included in herpes zoster shingles treatment. Antiviral drugs are specifically built to target viruses, stop their development, and sometimes even deactivate them. While no antiviral drug can eliminate the Varicella-Zoster Virus, there are some drugs that can stop the virus from replicating, thereby **reducing the duration of herpes zoster shingles**. Treatment using antiviral drugs can reduce the duration and severity of herpes zoster, provided a 7-10-day course of these drugs is started within 72 hours of the appearance of the characteristic shingles rash.

The standard antiviral for the Varicella-Zoster virus is Acyclovir. It has a long history of successfully treating herpetic viruses and its developer, Gertrude B. Elion, was awarded the Noble Prize for Medicine in 1988. Although acyclovir is quite effective against the Varicella-Zoster virus, it can also have some adverse effects. The most common adverse effects of acyclovir are nausea, vomiting, diarrhea and headaches. Other, more severe effects have also been known to happen with acyclovir, but only in less than 0.1% of the patients. These include coma, seizures, fatigue, anorexia, crystalluria, neutropenia, leucopenia and others.

Nowadays, although acyclovir is still the standard antiviral for Varicella-Zoster virus, there are two, more effective options available. Famciclovir and Valaciclovir are chemical derivatives of acyclovir and have demonstrated superiority in safety, efficacy and even tolerability. They also have another major advantage that recommends them over acyclovir. Famciclovir and Valaciclovir cannot only be used in the acute phase of the illness, but also as a method of prophylaxis. Note that antiviral treatments should only be used on patients with healthy immune systems. Serious complications can appear in patients that have their immune system compromised. The only way to minimize the risks of complications in these cases is to administer acyclovir intravenously. Although hard evidence has not been demonstrated that acyclovir can produce teratogenic or carcinogenic effects, treatment with acyclovir during pregnancy should be avoided as a precaution, because it can act as a chromosomal mutagen. Treatment with an antiviral during a pregnancy should only be considered if the effects of the shingles disease are acute. If the pain is extreme, or the rash is severe, an antiviral should only be prescribed in the later stages of the pregnancy, as the risks to the fetus will decrease by then.

Corticosteroids

Along with an antiviral, prednisone can also help reduce the healing time. Prednisone is a corticosteroid used to suppress the immune system. The combination of prednisone and acyclovir has had dramatic results with patients over 50 years of age. Some studies have shown that this combination can reduce the time it takes the blisters to form a crust by up to 50%, and lead to a significant decrease in the chances of the patient developing post herpetic neuralgia. However, the risks associated with corticosteroid treatments are high. Side effects are numerous and can be extremely severe; these include adrenal insufficiency, anovulation, menstrual irregularity, growth failure, glaucoma, cataracts, hyperglycemia, osteoporosis, extreme weight gain and others. Due to the risks of these treatments, they are only recommended in patients over the age of 50. This is mainly due to the greatly increased risk of post herpetic neuralgia, which increases when the patient is over 50 years of age.

Medication side effects and Natural Remedies

The side effects of herpes zoster shingles medication can be frightening. If the patient is not comfortable or is scared of taking drugs, there are a few natural remedies available. Natural remedies have a less impressive efficacy rate, but they do not come with the many possible side effects of conventional medicines.

There are some natural remedies available, which can act as an antiviral, an anti-septic and even as an anti-neuralgic. Natural remedies should be used by patients with a high degree of risk to the adverse effects of a chemical antiviral, analgesic or anti-septic. People with compromised immune systems, pregnant women and other patients that suffer from a second condition (other than herpes zoster shingles) should definitely see a medical specialist before resorting to natural remedies. Some of these natural remedies are provided in the next section.

In clinical practice, a commonly used treatment flowchart is usually followed. The following figure outlines the usual treatment course when a patient presents with Herpes zoster Shingles.

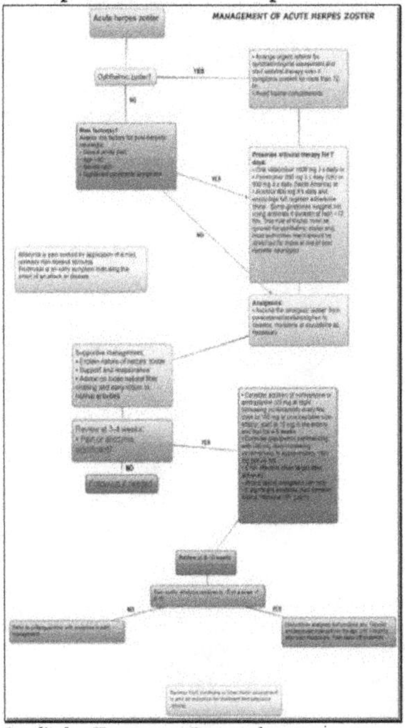

Credit for Treatment Protocols:

Management of Acute Herpes Zoster. International Herpes Management Forum treatment recommendations for herpes zoster and post-herpetic neuralgia. Diagram courtesy of Dr. Robert W.

Johnson, University of Bristol and Bristol Royal Infirmary, Bristol, UK. Adapted from "Management of PHN in the Immunocompetent Patient", Herpes 10:2, 2003.

6 How to Manage Shingles

Herpes Zoster Shingles is a common ailment for men and women, but that does not make it easier to manage. The pain can sometimes be intense, the medication can have drastic side effects, and the shingles rash can be very difficult to hide, making a herpes zoster shingles patient feel embarrassed when he or she mingles in society. Depression often accompanies this disease.

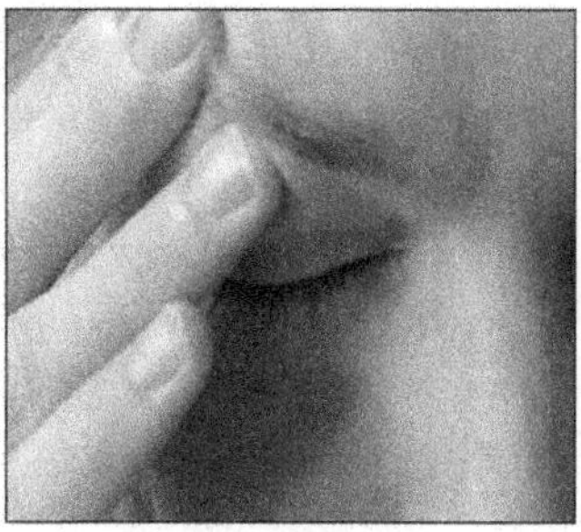

Pain management

The first thing a herpes zoster shingles patient has to deal with is the unrelenting pain that does not cease, day or night. Herpes zoster shingles patients often suffer from insomnia, because of this debilitating pain. The first step towards getting rid of herpes zoster shingles pain is to go to the doctor and get an analgesic prescribed. Lidocaine, calamine or capsaicin cream should be applied only on the affected rash areas. The frequency of the treatment depends upon the analgesic in use. **Capsaicin cream** should be used 3 to 5 times per day, while **lidocaine** can be applied as needed, with a minimum application interval of four hours. If the pain is too severe, narcotic medication (like morphine) should be used. However, this type of medication has serious side effects and patients will often suffer from anxiety attacks. To reduce the risk of anxiety and increase pain control, this type of analgesic should not be taken "as needed"; instead, regular doses should be the method of choice. Calamine and lidocaine should be used when the rash lesions are still open. Once a crust has formed (but not before) the patient should switch to the more powerful (and riskier) capsaicin cream.

Alternative Remedies

While prescription medications can be used to treat shingles blisters, they can result in sometimes harmful side effects. Many natural alternatives are available that effectively treat shingles without causing unnecessary harm. Some surprisingly effective home remedies are known, as a way to treat shingles blisters, and shingles pain. Several simple steps are shown here, using readily available ingredients. Since herpes zoster is a contagious virus, you should always wear gloves when applying a cream or placing a cloth over an infected individual's blisters.

First Step

Some over-the-counter hydrocortisone creams, such as Calamine lotion, Neosporin, or an oral antihistamine such as Benadryl, can relieve shingles-induced itching.

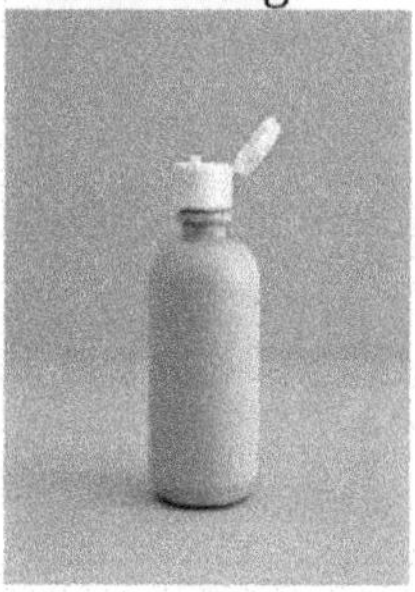

Calamine Lotion

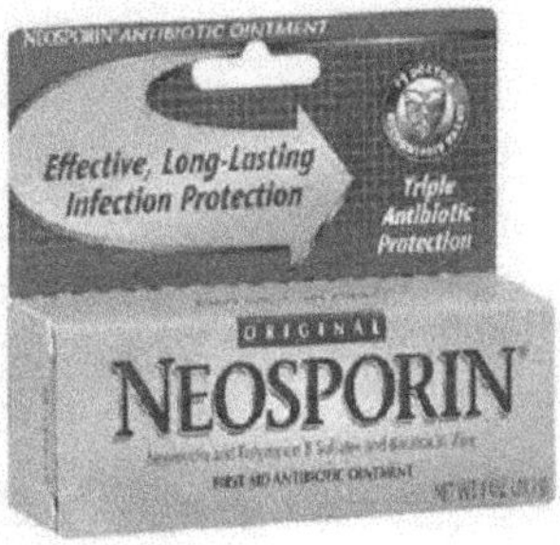

Neosporin

Second step

Mix an ounce of vinegar with 4 cups of cold water and then, use clean towels to make a cool compress. Apply a cool compress to the skin three times a day.

Third Step

Wash shingles blisters twice a day with soap and warm water so as to eliminate dirt that may cause skin irritation.

Fourth Step

Use a cream which contains capsaicin. Capsaicin reduces the presence of substance P, a neurochemical pain transmitter.

Fifth Step

Take a cool bath. Mix into the bath water some baking soda, raw oatmeal flakes, or colloidal oatmeal such as Aveeno. Or purchase an Aveeno bath over the counter.

Sixth Step

Eat the pineapple of the papaya fruit. Papaya fruits contain proteolytic enzymes, which are known to reduce inflammation.

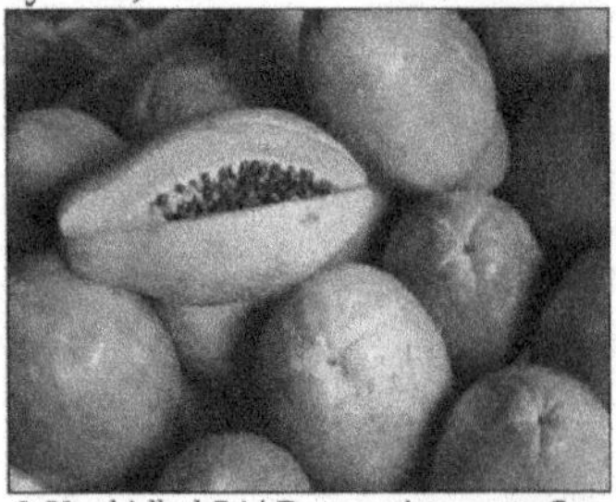

© Koakidbob54 | Dreamstime.com **Strawberry papayas**

While several prescription medications are available for the treatment of shingles, natural remedies are gentler and less likely to cause side effects. Try any of these natural remedies for shingles blisters and get instant relief safely and naturally.

Licorice

Licorice is a popular anti-viral herb that also contains compounds that boost the immune system. One can make an effective shingles remedy that can be applied directly to shingles blisters. A strong tea can be made by adding 3 to 4 sticks of licorice root (pictured below) to 1 cup of hot water, then allow this tea to steep for about 15 minutes. Soak a clean cloth in the liquid and then place this cloth directly to the shingles blisters for immediate shingles relief.

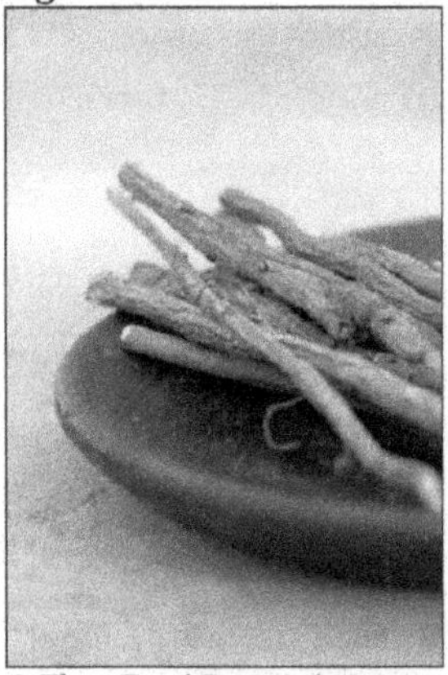

© Elena Ray | Dreamstime.com **Licorice root**

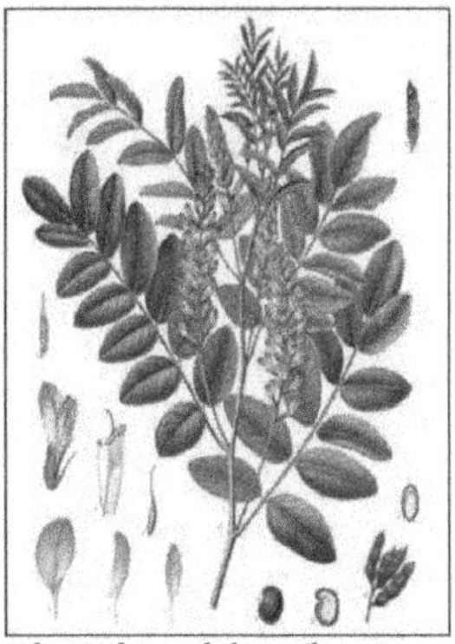

Glycyrrhiza glabra, (licorice root) from Franz Eugen Köhler, *Köhler's Medizinal-Pflanzen*

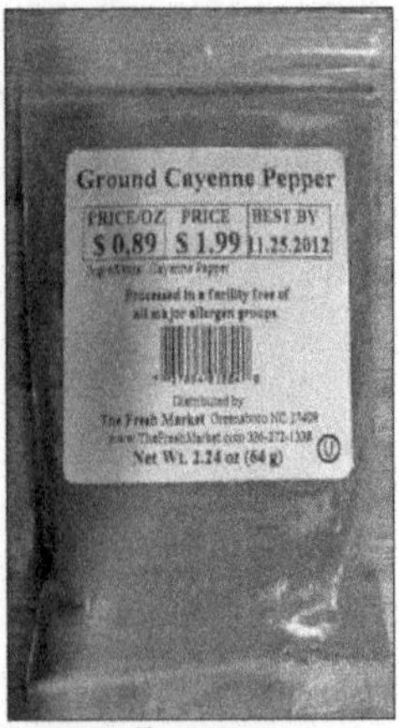

Cayenne Pepper

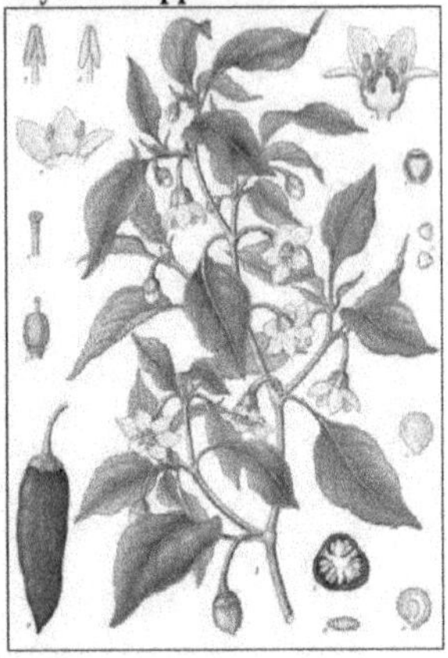

Cayenne Pepper

Capsicum annuum, from Franz Eugen Köhler, *Köhler's Medizinal-Pflanzen*

Cayenne pepper contains the active ingredient capsaicin, which prevents nerves under the skin from sending pain signals. This makes capsaicin one of the most effective home remedies for shingles. However, because of its strength, it should be combined with a white skin lotion. Mix small amounts of powdered cayenne pepper with two tablespoons of lotion until the lotion becomes a pinkish color. Then, apply a small amount of the lotion to some healthy skin, to see if any irritation occurs. If it does, add more lotion to the mixture, thereby diluting the capsaicin concentration, and try again. Lastly, rub this lotion directly into the shingles blisters to block pain and grant immediate shingles relief.

Lemon Balm

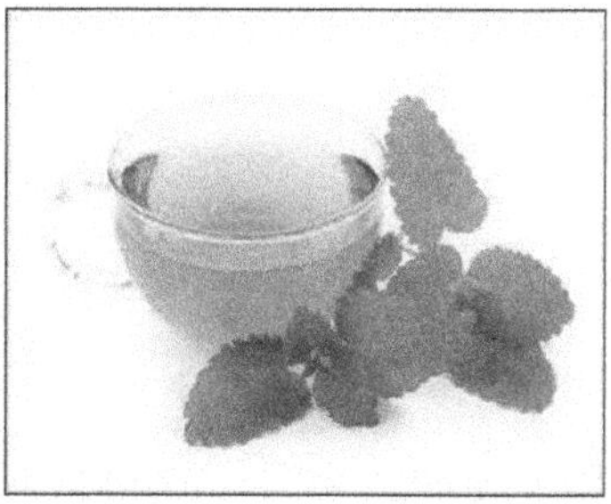

© Elena Schweitzer | Dreamstime.com **Lemon Balm Tea**
Citrus limon, from Franz Eugen Köhler,
Köhler'sMedizinal-Pflanzen

Lemon balm is an herb in the mint family, and has been found to be effective in treating viral infections. A tea made from dried lemon balm can be directly applied to the shingles blisters to reduce irritation and inflammation. To make the tea, combine two teaspoons of dried lemon balm with a cup of boiling water and allow this mixture to steep for about 15 minutes. Strain out the lemon balm, and then allow this tea to cool down to room temperature. Then, soak a clean cloth in the tea and apply this cloth directly to the shingles blisters. Do this several times a day to provide natural relief from shingles.

Turmeric

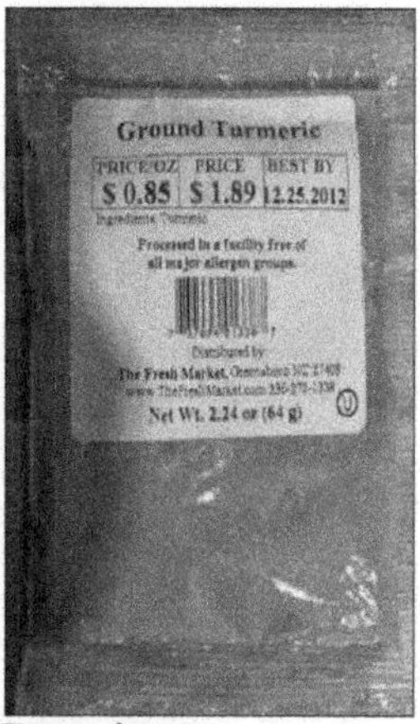

Turmeric

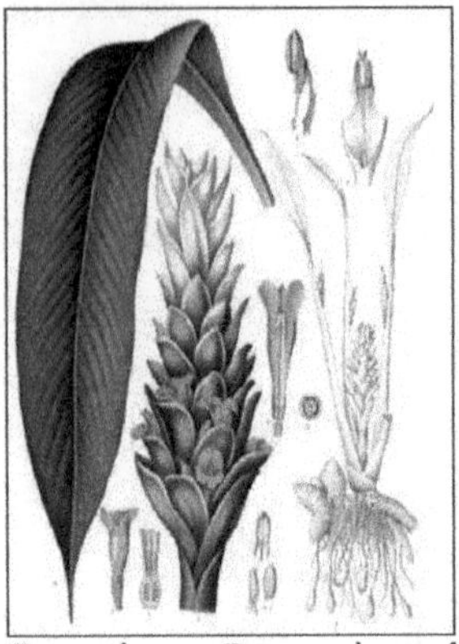

Turmeric *Curcuma longa,* from Franz Eugen Köhler, *Köhler's Medizinal-Pflanzen*

Using 3 tablespoons of turmeric, and 3 cups of water, bring turmeric and water to a boil. Let this mixture boil around 10 minutes until it forms a thick paste. If needed, add more water. Once the mixture starts to thicken slightly, you must stir it constantly to prevent scorching. Store the turmeric paste in a glass jar in a refrigerator. Then, apply the turmeric paste directly to the blister area, cover lightly with gauze. This will help dry the blisters up and accelerate the healing process. For shingles, an ayurvedic remedy calls for first spreading a light coating of mustard oil on the shingles rash, and then spreading the turmeric paste over that.

Using Turmeric, make a paste from the powder. To the blistered area of the skin, apply this paste for pain relief, and to speed healing.

Garlic

Finally, remember that garlic is good for infections and combating virus.

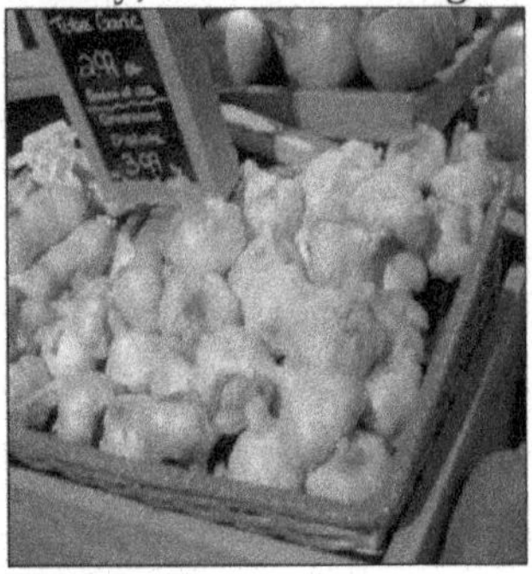

Garlic

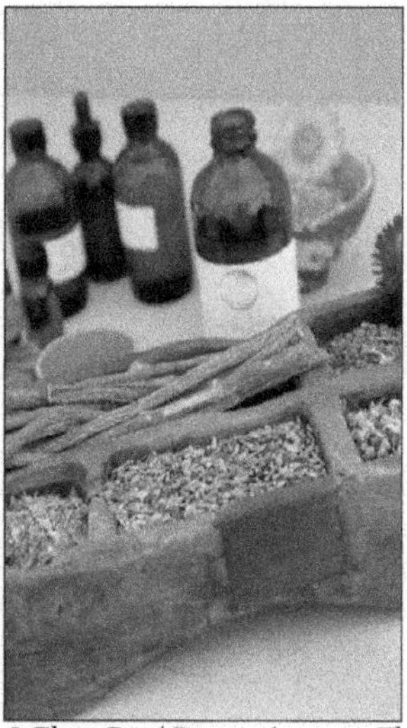

© Elena Ray | Dreamstime.com The holistic ingredients of Ayurveda and Herbalism including licorice root, milk thistle seeds, valerian root, chamomile, and tincture bottles.

Essential Oils

Many essential oils are available for shingles. They can be directly applied directly to shingles blisters to provide fast relief. These essential oils include bergamot, chamomile, geranium, lavender, eucalyptus, tea tree oil and lemon, among others. One can purchase essential oils at natural health stores. Essential oils are quite powerful; they must be diluted before application. Typically, one adds two to three drops of a particular essential oil to two tablespoons of vegetable oil, and then applies this mixture directly to a shingles blister. Be careful; never consume any essential oils as they can cause serious illness or even death if taken internally. As an example of how powerful essential oils can be in remedying shingles, consider the combination of ravensara and calophyllum:

The Essential Oils Desk Reference (Essential Science Publishing, 2009) states: "Equal amounts of Ravensara and Calophyllum inophyllum applied to a shingles outbreak have produced dramatic improvement and complete remission within 7 days" (see Alternative Medicine, The Definitive Guide, -. 56, 971).

Ravensara aromatica (also called *clove nutmeg*) is a member of the laurel tree family, which comes from Madagascar. The leaves and twigs of *R. aromatica* have a mildly camphorous aroma similar to eucalyptus. This essential oil has antiseptic, antibacterial, anti-viral and anti-infective properties. Calophyllum is a large evergreen tree, native to East Africa, and southern coastal India.

The Raindrop Technique

A somewhat controversial technique, pioneered by Gary Young, N.D. is presented at:

Raindrop Technique – the Essential Oil Massage for Aching Backs and Sore Muscles

According to this technique and website,

"'The Raindrop Technique uses clinically tested essential oils that have antiviral, antibacterial, and anti-inflammatory properties and are soothing and energizing to the body, as well. Raindrop is so powerful because it helps bring the body's systems into alignment.'

"Where Did The Technique Come From?

This innovative technique originated from the research of D. Gary Young N.D. and an idea he got from a Lakota medicine man named Wallace Black Elk over two decades ago. It combines Vita Flex (similar to reflexology) and specific massage techniques with therapeutic-grade essential oils to bring the body into structural and electrical alignment.

Why Is It Called Raindrop?

Raindrop got its name because the oils are dispensed like little drops of rain, from a height of about six to twelve inches. The oils are then gently massaged alongside the vertebrae with a "feathering" motion inspired by Lakota techniques.

The Raindrop Technique uses 9 essential oils: 7 single oils and 2 therapeutic blends. After the essential oils have been applied, a steam heated towel is placed on the back for 10 to 15 minutes, allowing the recipient to relax deeper. (Patients with certain conditions, such as MS, have a cold towel applied instead of a hot towel.)

How Long Does It Take?

The entire Raindrop process takes about 50 – 60 minutes to complete. Although it takes less than an hour, the oils will continue working in the body for several days.

What Can Raindrop Can Do For Me?

Obviously, Raindrop is a deeply relaxing, aromatic and pleasurable experience. For that alone, it is very much worth the experience.

In addition, therapeutic-grade essential oils stimulate (or 'wake-up') your body's natural healing response. Because they are so multi-faceted and complex, they connect with your body's innate intelligence. Their holistic action encourages your body to heal not only on the physical level, but on the mental, emotional, and spiritual levels as well.

The therapeutic-grade essential oils used in Raindrop also stimulate the body to begin releasing toxins."

Antivirals to the rescue, and their side effects

Shingles cases need to be treated as early as possible. Three antiviral agents can effectively deal with herpes zoster shingles: **acyclovir, famciclovir and valacyclovir**. When dealing with the Varicella-Zoster virus, acyclovir is the bread and butter antiviral. A DNA polymerase inhibitor, acyclovir can be delivered in two ways, orally or intravenously. Just like acyclovir, famciclovir is also a DNA polymerase inhibitor but it is a more recently developed drug, and it has some advantages over acyclovir. The dosage is the first advantage; with acyclovir, a patient will usually take five doses every day for about seven to ten days, while famciclovir is usually taken three times per day. That is also the case with valacyclovir, which should be taken three times per day. Another advantage for valacyclovir and famciclovir is that their bioavailability is much better than that of acyclovir.

The choice of an antiviral depends upon each person. Each antiviral has equivalent side effects and the relative difference among these antivirals is not large. Along with an antiviral, a doctor will often prescribe corticosteroids such as prednisone. Results when using corticosteroids vary, but physicians are sure that it helps patients who are over the age of 50 decreases the chances of neuralgia, and it helps reduce the herpes zoster shingles pain. The corticosteroid dosage usually starts at 30 mg and the dosage gradually decreases as the treatment progresses. The treatment for patients with ocular shingles is nearly the same. Antivirals and corticosteroids are used in these cases.

Preventive treatment?

Unfortunately, a safe preventive treatment for shingles has not been developed yet. It is unlikely that a patient, who has safely been treated for herpes zoster shingles, will develop the sickness again. Dealing with shingles usually provides immunologic protection, but if the patient's immune system is compromised, the Varicella-Zoster virus may reactivate itself, and one needs to recognize this outcome may appear.

7 Dietary Approaches to Shingles Treatment

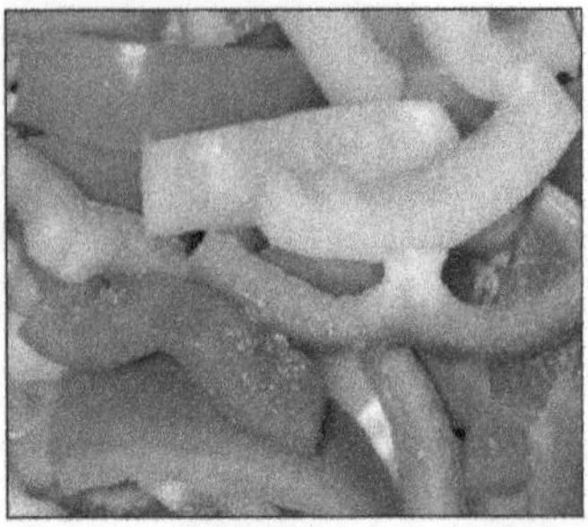

Having a good diet enhances our immune system, and herpes zoster shingles is no exception. With a well balanced diet, your body gets all the nutrients it needs to better fight the disease. Also, take a Vitamin B supplement to boost your immunity.

In the case of herpes zoster shingles, vegetables and fruits work best. In particular, eat a lot of papayas and pineapple to improve immunity. These are rich in vitamins, which help a patient's immune system fight the virus. Any fruit that is rich in vitamin C will enhance one's immune system. The importance of a strong immune system cannot be stressed enough. Not only will your immune system help the body fight the virus, but also it can help in preventing a future outbreak of herpes zoster shingles.

One should try to keep your diet as natural as possible when trying to fight herpes zoster shingles. When receiving a treatment for herpes zoster shingles, there may be several dietary restrictions. For example, when taking corticosteroids, one should reduce sodium intake (salt) as much as possible. In addition, a person on corticosteroids should refrain from eating spicy foods, sweets, heavy food, or sodas. One should keep their diet as clean and as light as possible, and drink lots of water, as it helps purify the body.

While suffering from herpes zoster shingles, a patient must be careful with food. Almost any treatment for shingles has culinary restrictions. Some foods are spiced with additives, which might interfere with herpes zoster shingles treatment. For example, if one eats food containing sodium (salt, potatoes, radishes and others) while on corticosteroids, the body will retain this sodium. Sodium's main function in the human body is to cause water retention. Therefore, upon ingestion, the patient will start retaining water, get bloated, gain weight and the body will not respond as well to treatment.

Treatment complications due to improper diet

When on a treatment for shingles, always check the medication prescription for any counter-indications and obey the physician's words to the letter. As long as a patient respects the drug prescription and the doctor's orders, he or she will find that herpes zoster shingles is not difficult to handle. As long as one does not slip up, the chances for complications will be minimal. A poor diet will only lengthen healing time with a shingles drug treatment.

8 Shingles Complications

Herpes zoster shingles is a disease that can have very serious complications. Some complications happen because of the nature of the disease, some occur because of the place where the rash is localized, and

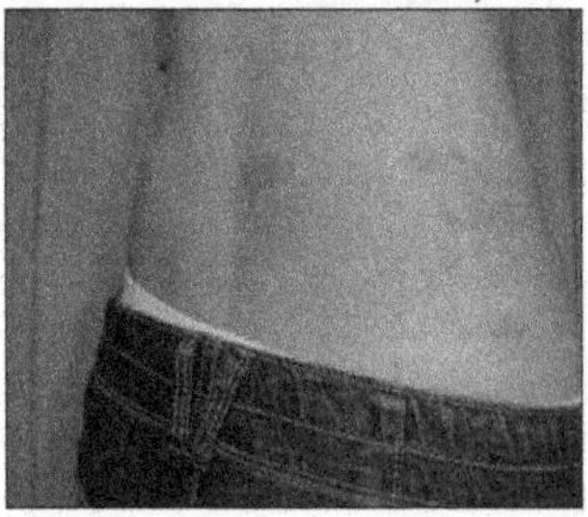

others occur because of the treatment itself.

There are several complications to herpes zoster shingles; some of them happen frequently, while others have a very slim chance of materializing. Here are some of the most common herpes zoster shingles complications:

Post-Herpetic Neuralgia

This is the most common complication of herpes zoster shingles. Post-herpetic neuralgia (PHN) occurs when the shingles rash has disappeared, but the shingles pain does not stop. It is caused by damage to the neuron from the zoster virus. It has a higher incidence for patients that are over 50 years of age, but it also happens to younger patients. The pain can be mild to severe, and even excruciating in the most severe of cases. Post-herpetic neuralgia can last from weeks to years. There is no cure for PHN, so the only option is to try to **treat the symptoms**. In the extreme cases, post herpetic neuralgia can have complications of its own. The most common of these are insomnia, disability, depression and weight loss. It is not difficult to understand these complications, because it can be extremely hard on a patient's psyche to withstand dealing with that amount of pain, with no certainty when the shingles will go away. Fortunately, a patient has many options concerning medication, which can help deal with the pain.

There are four major medication categories, which can be used for post-herpetic neuralgia relief:

The first category is **tricyclic antidepressants**. This is the most commonly used when dealing with post herpetic neuralgia. The most common tricyclic antidepressant used is amitryptiline. While it may be quite effective, it has many negative side effects. Newer treatments include drugs with considerably less side effects like desipramine and nortriptyline. Due to their complications and side effects, tricyclic antidepressants should not be used by patients with heart problems or narrow angle glaucoma.

Anticonvulsants make up the second category of drugs for post herpetic neuralgia. These are medications used for treating seizures and pain. The most commonly prescribed anticonvulsant, when dealing with post herpetic neuralgia, is gabapentin. Its side effects are rare and mild, so it is an excellent option for elderly patients with PHN.

The third category of drugs is used for the extreme cases of post-herpetic neuralgia. These are the opioids. An extremely strong pain medication, opioids will most likely be effective in lessening any form of pain. Unfortunately, opiods also have a narcotic effect and can be highly addictive. The most common opioids used for post herpetic neuralgia are morphine, methadone, oxycodone and tramadol. These can have very strong side effects and should never be used on patients with a history of addiction.

The fourth and last category of drugs is the topical local anesthetics. This type of medication is also used during the herpes zoster shingles disease and it usually comes in the form of a cream, lotion or spray that the patient applies on the affected areas. The most commonly used topical local anesthetics are lidocaine and capsaicin.

Post-Herpetic Itch

Post herpetic itch might not seem like much of a complication at first, but sometimes it can be even more difficult to manage than post herpetic neuralgia. Post-herpetic itch patients are advised not to scratch, because this can lead to injury and even infections. It is very difficult to treat; the only types of medication, which have had some success, are the topical local anesthetics, and only those, which numb the skin.

Herpes Zoster *ophthalmicus* Complications

The Herpes zoster shingles condition is considered herpes zoster *ophthalmicus* when the affected area is located near the eye or is in the eye itself. In this case, complications can be extremely severe. From eye infection to immediate loss of sight, complications are common with herpes zoster ophthalmicus. If a patient develops herpes zoster *ophthalmicus*, he should see an ophthalmologist immediately. There is no special treatment for it, but the ophthalmologist may find it necessary to prescribe some medication, which can protect the patient's eyes. Shown below is a typical case of herpes zoster *ophthalmicus*.

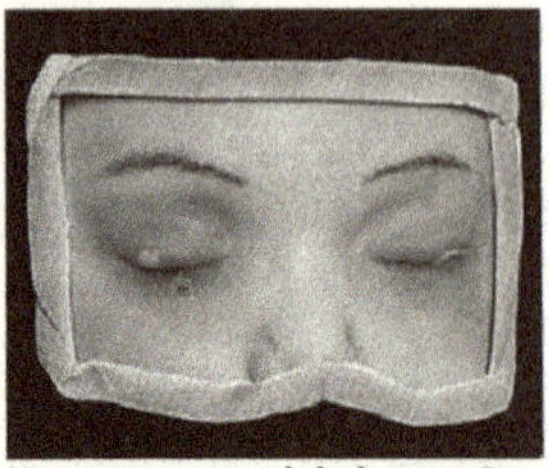

Herpes zoster *ophthalmicus*. Images courtesy *Atlas of external diseases of the eye*, By Richard Greeff, Rebman Company, N.Y., 1914.

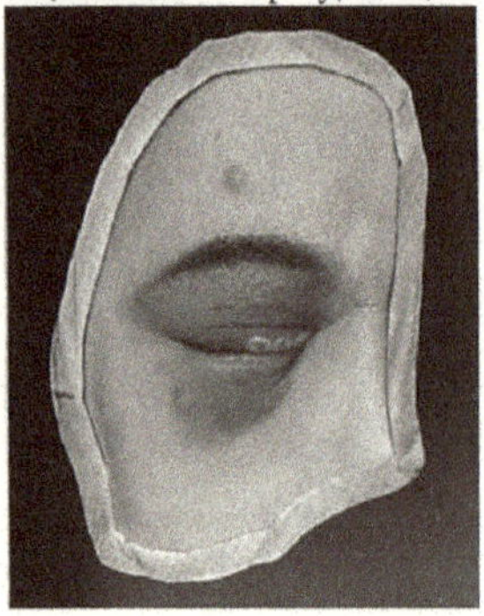

Ramsay Hunt Syndrome

Ramsay Hunt syndrome is a complication of herpes zoster shingles, when it is located near or within the ear. This condition is also called Herpes Zoster *oticus*. Patients affected will suffer from hearing disorders and severe loss of balance. In addition, loss of control over the facial muscles is common with this complication. In the most severe cases, Ramsay Hunt syndrome can affect a person's central nervous system (the brain and spinal cord). This is one of the most severe shingles developments, as the mortality rate in such cases is quite high. Stroke or meningitis is likely to occur if a patient's central nervous system becomes involved. In the following two images, an individual is shown with peripheral facial palsy in conjunction with an eruption of Herpes Zoster *oticus*.

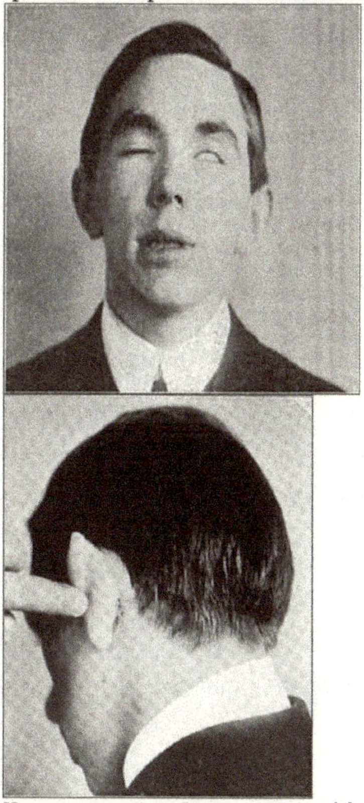

Herpes zoster *oticus*. Images courtesy of the Archives of Internal Medicine, Vol. V, 1910, the American Medical Association

Bacterial Infections

Bacterial infections are common with shingles patients that have itchy rashes. Because the patient tends to scratch, the blisters frequently break, and provide an easy entrance route for bacteria. The only way to prevent this from happening is to completely refrain from scratching the affected area. Bacterial infections are treated with antibiotics, as the patient's doctor sees fit.

Complications with Herpes Zoster Shingles and Pregnancy

Shingles complications with pregnancy vary, depending on the progress of the pregnancy when the infection occurs. If a pregnant mother becomes infected while in the first four months of pregnancy, there will be some risk of congenital malformations. If the infection occurs just before birth (20 to 5 days before), the risk of the baby contracting chickenpox is almost 100%. Such cases can sometimes be lethal, because a newborn's immune system is not developed. Therefore, it has almost no protection against the virus. The only treatment is a transfusion of immune globulin from a patient, which has recently had herpes zoster shingles. Therefore, the blood is rich with antibodies.

Complications of Herpes Zoster Shingles Treatment

Shingles treatment complications are directly linked to the type of treatment the patient has received. These usually include side effects from medication and the conditions that develop if the patient does not observe the counter-indications. These complications vary from person to person and can be mild to severe.

Note that all of these complications are more likely to happen with patients having a compromised immune system. If a patient's immune system is compromised, the chances of complications increase greatly. For HIV patients, or patients who have been treated with an immunosuppressant agent, herpes zoster shingles can be deadly.

9 Is there a Shingles Vaccine?

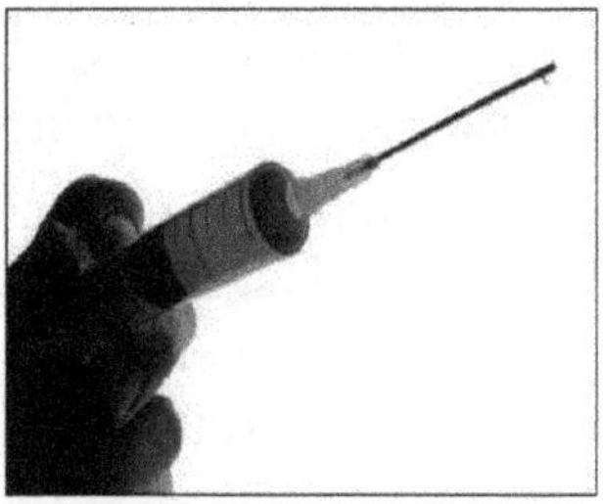

The FDA approved **Zostavax®** from Merck (Live Zoster Vaccine) in 2006 for use in adults **ages 60 and over** who have had chickenpox. In 2006, the Advisory Committee on Immunization Practices recommended immunizing everyone over 60 years of age with a history of chickenpox. This is in addition to the previously used vaccine against chickenpox (Varivax®) used for children that are older than 18 months.

In prior clinical research, a double-blind study was performed and results were very positive. In a population size of over 38,000 senior citizens, the number of Herpes zoster shingles cases was reduced by more than 50%. In addition, many patients, who developed herpes zoster shingles, displayed symptoms that were considerably milder, the recovery time was decreased, and the number of complications was dramatically reduced. Note that the vaccine is useless in patients that are currently suffering from Herpes zoster shingles. It is only a means of preventing shingles, not a way to treat or cure it. If a patient is already suffering from Herpes zoster shingles or chickenpox, the use of a vaccine against shingles is not recommended. The reason why the shingles vaccine is approved only for the age category of 50+ years is because of the prevalence of shingles in this age category. This is the group most likely to get shingles. Few people under 50 get shingles, so a vaccine to address younger age groups is not cost effective. Protection from the shingles vaccine lasts at least six years.

For your reference, a **shingles vaccine information statement** is included in the appendix.

10 Conclusions

Since the 18th century, when William Heberden found a way to differentiate smallpox and herpes zoster shingles, mankind has tried to find a treatment for shingles. Now, in the 21th century, we are closer to finding answers to a cure for this disease. With several major health agencies doing research worldwide, herpes zoster shingles may go the way of smallpox in the future. With shingles as contagious as it is, public health education and research towards destroying this virus is important.

Patients with Herpes zoster shingles consider themselves unlucky, without knowing that it is a very common affliction. Hundreds of thousands of people get sick with shingles every year, and they are treated, usually with minimal complications. The first step in overcoming Herpes zoster shingles is keeping a positive mindset, and not panicking. As you have seen in this report, there are a wide variety of ways to treat your case of shingles. The medical research effort has paid off with an impressive set of antivirals and analgesics. On the other hand, alternative medicine, ayurvedic medicine and traditional healing methods have also provided a variety of helpful remedies.

A new understanding of the molecular basis of VZV and its associated encoded gene products my eventually allow recombinant vaccines or specifically designed antibody therapies that may permit novel therapeutic approaches. Ultimately, shingles may be completely preventable.

11 Frequently Asked Questions about Shingles

Question: How long does a shingles outbreak typically last?

Answer: shingles will last 3 to 4 weeks from start to finish

Question: If you have had chickenpox, can you catch shingles from someone else?

Answer: No, by having chickenpox, an individual already has a population of dormant VZV in their body.

Question: Is shingles contagious?

Answer: Yes, shingles is contagious. The virus that causes shingles is a member of the herpes virus family. An individual can become infected by exposure to someone with shingles, and then develop chickenpox.

Question: Can I give shingles to others?

Answer: No one can get shingles from you. However, you can transmit the chickenpox virus to other individuals. Exercise caution and refrain from exposing others to your shingles rash.

Question: Is shingles related to chickenpox?

Answer: Shingles is a rash of the skin caused by the same herpes zoster virus that causes chickenpox.

Question: Can a person with chickenpox transmit shingles to someone else?

Answer: No, a person can communicate the Varicella Zoster virus, but this will only transmit chickenpox to an uninfected individual, not shingles.

Question: What percentage of people who have had chickenpox will get shingles?

Answer: About 20 percent of the population

Question: Once you get shingles, will you get it again?

Answer: The majority of people get shingles only once in their lifetime. Some individuals can, however, get shingles again.

Question: What do doctors perform to reach a diagnosis of shingles?

Answer: Physicians do a laboratory diagnosis of the shingles blister fluid, and also a visual diagnosis of the patient, to confirm a diagnosis of shingles.

Question: Is permanent scarring left after a shingles outbreak?

Answer: Usually, no scarring is left when the blisters disappear.

Question: How long do shingles blisters last?

Answer: Shingles blisters normally remain from 1 to 14 days

Question: Is there a cure for shingles?

Answer: There is no cure. Medical research is actively pursuing a cure.

Recently, a shingles vaccine has been developed for individuals over the age of 60.

Question: Who is doing shingles research?

Answer: The National Institute of Neurological Disorders and Stroke (NINDS) and other institutes of the National Institutes of Health (NIH), among others

Question: Where in the body does the Varicella Zoster virus (VZV) settle in?

Answer: In the dorsal nerve roots and ganglia

Question: Is shingles caused by the same herpes virus responsible for genital herpes?

Answer: The genital herpes virus is not the same as the Varicella Zoster virus that causes shingles and chickenpox.

Question: What are the symptoms and signs of shingles?

Answer: Oozing blisters or pain without blisters, burning pain and sensitive skin, on one side of the body. Shingles appears as a rash on **one side of the back, chest, face and/or legs**. This is because the zoster virus follows a nerve pathway and nerves do not cross the midline of the body

Question: What is the most common complication of shingles?

Answer: Nerve pain (post herpetic neuralgia or PHN)

Question: If you have never had chickenpox, and you are over age 60, should you take the shingles vaccine Zostavax?

Answer: No, see the Vaccine Information sheet for shingles.

Question: At what age is the shingles vaccine available?

Answer: Zostavax is approved for adults age 60 or over

Question: Can people with a weak immune system, who do not have the zoster virus, get this virus from a person who has shingles?

Answer: Yes, the weaker the immune system, the more likelihood a person has to contract the VZV

Shingles Health Organizations

American Chronic Pain Association (ACPA)
Email: ACPA@pacbell.net

http://www.theacpa.org

P.O. Box 850
Rocklin, CA 95677-0850

Tel: 916-632-0922 800-533-3231

Fax: 916-652-8190

National Shingles Foundation [For Research on Varicella Zoster]
Email: vzv@vzvfoundation.org

http://www.vzvfoundation.org

603 W. 115 Street

Suite 371

New York, NY 10025

Tel: 212-222-3390
Fax: 212-838-0380

References

Oxford, J.S. and Oberg, B. Conquest of viral diseases: a topical review of drugs and vaccines, 2003

Arvin, A.M., Varicella-zoster Virus, Springer-Verlag, 2010.

Davison, A.J. and Scott, J.E. The complete DNA sequence of varicella-zoster virus. *J. Gen. Virol*. 1986; 67: 2279-2286

Goodpasture, E.W., Anderson, K. Infection of human skin, grafted on the chorioallantois of chick embryos, with the virus of herpes zoster. *Am. J. Pathol*. 1944; 20: 447-455.

Head, H., Campbell, A.W. The pathology of herpes zoster and its bearing on sensory localization. *Brain* 1900; 23:353-523

Hope-Simpson, R.E. The nature of herpes zoster: a long-term study and a new hypothesis. *Proc. Royal Soc. Med.*, 1965; 58:9-20

Johnson, R.W. Herpes Zoster in the Immunocompetent Patient: Management of Post-herpetic Neuralgia, *Herpes* 10:2, 2003.

Kundratitz, K. Experimentelle Übertragung von Herpes Zoster auf den Menschen und die Beziehungen von Herpes Zoster zu Varicellen (in German). *Monatsschrift Kinderheillkd* 1925; 29:516-522.

Minarovitz J., Gonczol, E. and Valyi-Nagy, T. Latency Strategies of herpes viruses, 2007

Redman, R.L. Nader, S., Zerboni, L., et al. Early reconstitution of immunity and decreased severity of herpes zoster in bone marrow transplant recipients immunized with inactivated varicella vaccine. *J. Infect. Dis*. 1997; 176:578-585.

Takahishi, M., Otsuka, T, Okuno, Y, et al. Live vaccine used to prevent the spread of varicella in children in hospital. *Lancet* 1974; 2: 1288-1290.

Von Bokay, J. Über den ätiologischen Zussamenhang der Varizellen mit gewissen Fallen von Herpes-zoster, *Wien Klin Wochenschr*.1909; 22:1323-1326.

Weller, T.H., Stoddard, M.B. Intranuclear inclusion bodies in cultures of human tissue inoculated with varicella vesicle fluid. *J. Immunol* 1952; 68:311-319.

Wood, M.J. History of Varicella Zoster Virus, *Herpes* 7:3, 2000.

Appendix

Acyclovir – one of the most commonly used drugs for the treatment of Herpes Zoster Simplex infection. The drug is marketed under the names of Herpex, Acivir, Acivirax, Zovirax, Aciclovir, Zovir and Cyclovir. Some of the common side effects include diarrhea, nausea, vomiting, and headaches and in high doses hallucinations; other side effects experienced by some patients included vertigo, dizziness, sore throat, abdominal pain, hair loss, etc. (see chemical structure)

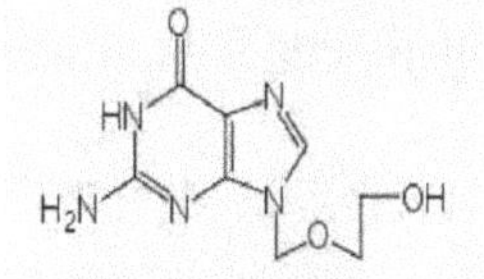

Adrenal insufficiency – condition in which the adrenal glands do not produce enough steroid hormones, causing a person to become dehydrated, disoriented, experience weakness, dizziness, nausea, vomiting and diarrhea.

Aerosols – technically, these are fine solid particles or liquid droplets in a gas or air.

Amitryptiline – this is a tricyclic antidepressant, one of the most widely used drugs for the treatment of depression. Some of the common side effects of this drug are drowsiness, weight gain, dry mouth, muscle stiffness, constipation, nausea, nervousness, urinary retention, blurred vision, insomnia and sexual function changes.

Antibiotics – simply put, these are substances that kill bacteria or slow their growth

Anticonvulsants –A wide group of drugs that are mainly used as mood stabilizers and to treat epileptic seizures. They work by suppressing the rapid and excessive firing of neurons that start a seizure.

Antiseptic – this is an antimicrobial substance, used on skin to reduce the possibility of infections, putrefaction or sepsis.

Anxiety attacks – also called panic attacks, are episodes of intense fear that have a fast onset and last for a small period – 10-30 minutes maximum. The shortest panic attacks last up to 15 seconds.

Calamine- mixture of zinc oxide with iron oxide, used as an anti-itching agent which is prescribed in the treatment of poison ivy, rashes, chickenpox and insect stings and bites.

Capsaicin – active compound of red hot chili peppers, medically used to treat and relieve post-herpetic neuralgia or peripheral neuropathy

Carcinogenic – wide name applied to any radiation, substance or radionuclide that is directly involved in causing cancer.

Cataracts – basically, a clouding over the crystalline lens of the eye; the degree of development varies from complete to slight opacity of the passage of light

Chickenpox - a disease common among young people, which manifests itself through virulent outbursts of itchy blisters all over the body

Conjunctivitis – this is an infection of the outermost layer of the eye (conjunctiva) and inner surface of the eyelids. Also called pink eye or madras eye.

Crystalluria – the crystals found in human urine (see figure)

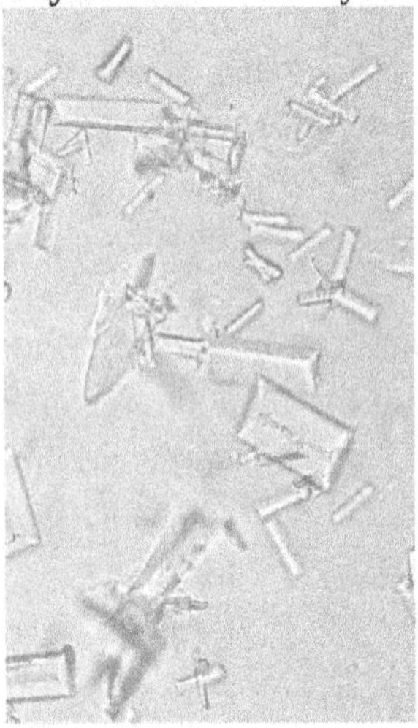

Desipramine – tricyclic antidepressant used in the treatment of depression and in the treatment of neuropathic pain.

Famciclovir - this is an antiviral used mainly in the treatment of shingles. Marketed under the name Famvir, its adverse side effects include mild to extreme stomach upset, headaches, mild fever. (See chemical structure)

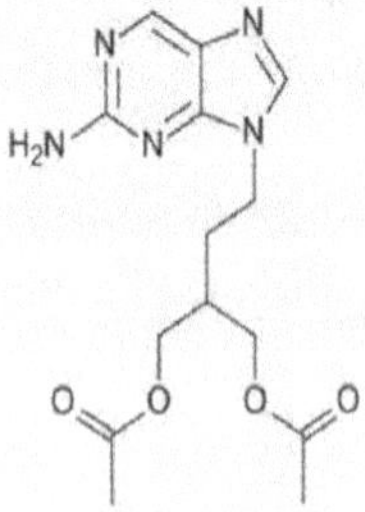

Gabapentin- a drug, branded as Neurontin, developed for the treatment of epilepsy that is currently used for the treatment of neuropathic pain.

Glaucoma – condition that manifests itself through an increase in fluid pressure inside the eye. This causes irreversible damage to the optic nerve, leading to vision loss.

Herpes zoster - aka shingles or zona, a viral disease that appears on the body as a rash that is very painful; blisters also occur.

Herpes zoster ophthalmicus – shingles infection located around the eye

Herpes zoster oticus – shingles infection located around the ear

Ibuprofen – an anti-inflammatory drug used to relieve symptoms of fever, dysmenorrhea, arthritis; the drug is also used as an analgesic (painkiller) and is marketed under various names.

IgM antibody – basic antibody present in the human system

Keratitis – disease in which the front part of the eye, the cornea, becomes inflamed. Moderate to intense pain are associated with this condition, and impaired eyesight follows.

Leucopenia – condition in which the white blood cell numbers decrease, placing the person at increased risk of getting infections

Lidocaine – common antiarrhythmic drug and local anesthetic, used to relieve itching, pain and burning from skin inflammations; also used as a local anesthetic for minor surgeries.

Lymph nodes – these are ball-shaped, small organs that are a part of the immune system; they are distributed widely throughout the body.

Morphine – a very potent analgesic made from opium, and considered the prototypical opioid. Highly addictive, withdrawal is very difficult. Used to treat all sorts of pain, withdrawal symptoms include anxiety, yawning, crying, cramping, involuntary muscle movements, insomnia, and elevated blood pressure. (See chemical structure)

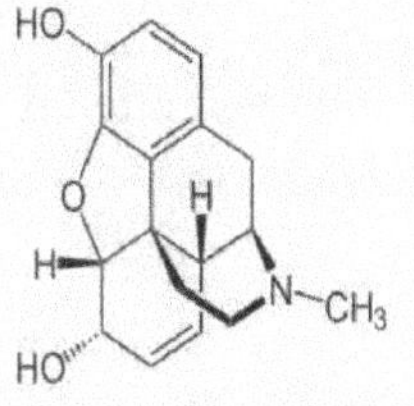

Neuralgia – nerve pain

Neutropenia - hematological disorder that is characterized by a very low number of neutrophils, these being the most important type of white blood cell in the human blood

Nortriptyline - is a tricyclic antidepressant used to treat major depression, bedwetting, and as an adjuvant in the treatment of chronic fatigue syndrome, migraine and chronic pain and other neurological conditions.

Opioids – they are the world's oldest drugs, used for their analgesic effects; side effects include addiction, sedation, constipation and respiratory depression

Osteoporosis – bone disease that leads to an increased risk of bone fractures

Oxycodone – opioid analgesic medication; side effects include memory loss, euphoria, fatigue, dizziness, constipation, nausea, headache, dry mouth, anxiety, pruritus and diaphoresis

Prednisone – a synthetic corticosteroid drug, used as an immunosuppressant. It has many side effects, and because it suppresses the immune system, it leaves patients vulnerable to infections.

Prophylaxis – preventive medicine, taking drugs to prevent the onset of diseases

Sensory ganglia – this is a nodule on a dorsal root that contains cell bodies of neurons in afferent spinal nerves.

Serous exudates – fluid that filters from the circulatory system into areas of inflammation or lesions.

Shingles - see Herpes Zoster

Tachycardia – accelerated heart rate

Teratogenic - the study of abnormalities of physiological development.

Tramadol – analgesic medication used in the treatment of mild to moderately severe pain

Tricyclic antidepressants – very commonly used antidepressants

Uveitis – severe inflammation of the middle layer of the eye that requires immediate medical attention as it can lead to blindness.

Valaciclovir – medication used in the treatment of herpes simplex and herpes zoster. The most common side effects include nausea, vomiting, diarrhea and headache. (See chemical structure)

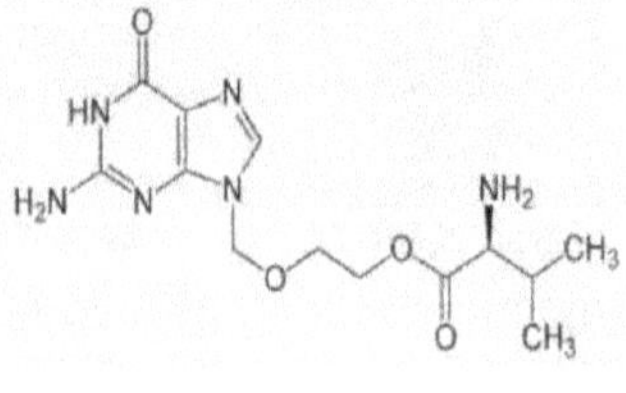

Varicella-Zoster Virus (VZV) - one of the

eight herpes viruses known to affect men, it is the main cause of chickenpox, shingles and post herpetic neuralgia.

Zoster sine herpete – See Herpes Zoster

CPSIA information can be obtained
at www.ICGtesting.com
Printed in the USA
LVHW091919251121
704460LV00003B/461

9 798740 456874